Skin care tips

Basic Skin Care Tips And Organic Facial Treatment

CONTENT

INTRODUCTION

Taking good care of your skin is important for more than just your appearance. As the largest organ you have, your skin is essential to your general health. If you take care of it, it can help take care of you. This is why it is so important to have a well thought out skin care routine. It is absolutely worth the time and energy to take care of your skin on daily basics, skin care is part of a healthy lifestyle.

Your skin health and you

Your skin health says a lot about you; your skin is the largest organ of your body and protector of everything that makes you. A healthy skin is an asset to the body; it helps regulate your body temperature, it acts as a natural filter of elements that affect your health, and it is constantly growing due to the rigorous and thankless jobs it is doing every day to keep you safe and healthy. Whatever you do; what you eat, what you drink, and the type of job you do, and the type of environment your body is exposed will have telling effects on your skin in good or bad ways.

<u>Why skin health all year round is important</u>
The sunburn in hot summer sun and the dry flaky skin in cold winter weather and the resulting discomforts should be a stern personal reminder of the importance of skin health all year round. Whether during a sunny or cold day your skin is affected one way or the other. Therefore, taking necessary skin health precautions will give you all year round protection against skin problems and if otherwise, may lead to more complications.

As the largest organ of your body, the skin plays the role of first line of defense in keeping you safe from infections and other unfriendly elements. It is for this reason that your skin needs to be in good health always. You should look good and also feel good inside.

CHAPTER ONE

Basic Steps On How To Take Good Take Care Of Your Skin

Wash your skin twice a day and whenever you sweat: Washing gets rid of oils, dirt, bacteria, and other nasty stuff that builds up on your skin throughout the day. Wash your face in the morning and evening to prevent clogged pores and breakouts.

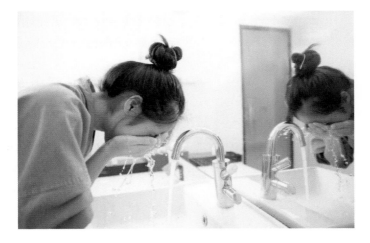

While dermatologists don't all agree on how often you should shower, most say it's a good idea to do it several times a week (e.g., every other day).

It's good to break a sweat sometimes, but letting sweat sit on your skin can cause acne breakouts and irritation.

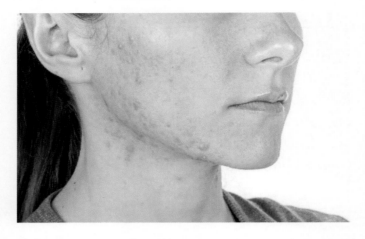

If it's hot out or you've been hitting the gym, change out of your sweaty clothes as soon as possible, take a shower, and wash your face.

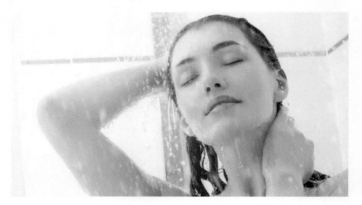

Wash any sweaty clothes before wearing them again. Wash up immediately after being in a swimming pool or in the ocean. If you wear makeup, wash it off every evening before you go to bed with an oil free makeup remover and a gentle cleanser.

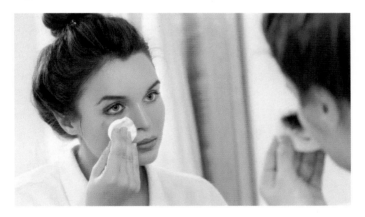

(Example of an oil free makeup remover)

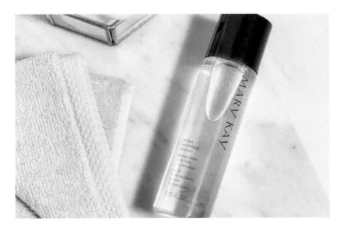

Cleanse yourself with warm water

Using hot water when you shower or wash your face can dry out and irritate your skin. Stick to washing with comfortably warm water instead.

Shorten your shower

Steam and heat can open pores and help you get rid of toxins. But running hot water over your skin for more than a few minutes at a time can strip away oil from your skin, leaving it looking tired and dull.

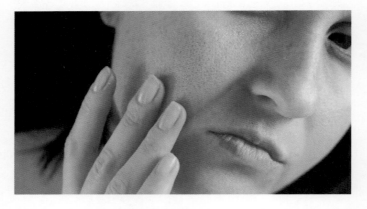

Try to minimize your skin's exposure to water that's extremely hot. You may also consider cooling down the temperature in the latter part of your shower to improve circulation, which may give your face a more toned and youthful appearance.

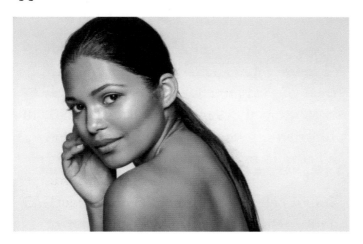

As an added benefit, this might even boost your immune system.

Apply your cleanser with your fingertips or a soft cloth:

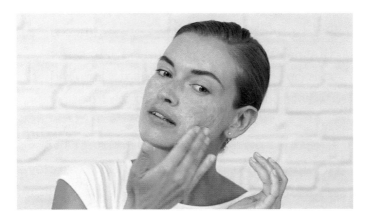

While exfoliating your skin occasionally can give it a healthy glow, regular scrubbing can cause irritation. Be kind to your face and wash it with your fingers instead of sponges or washcloths.

When you bath or shower, use a soft washcloth on your body if you want a little gentle exfoliation.

If you have a skin condition such as psoriasis,

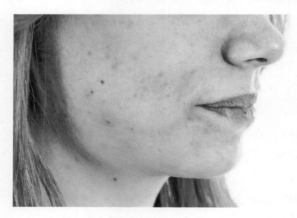

Don't use washcloths, loofahs, sponges, or scrub brushes. Stick to gently cleansing your skin with your hands.

Rinse off your cleanser thoroughly

When you're done Even a gentle cleanser can irritate your skin if you don't rinse it away when it away when you're done washing! Use warm water and your hands to gently rinse away any residue that's left on your skin.

If you like, you can rinse your face with cool water when you're done cleaning it. The cold temperatures will temporarily tighten up your skin and minimize the appearance of pores.

Pat your skin dry with a clean, dry towel

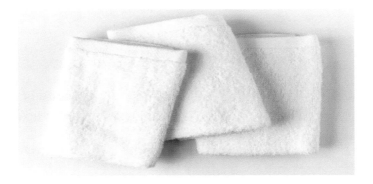

When you're done washing up, don't rub your skin with a towel, since this can be irritating. Instead, take a soft towel and blot or pat your skin to remove excess moisture. Your skin will thank you for the TLC!

If you have dry skin, apply a little moisturizer immediately after patting yourself dry, while your skin is still slightly damp.

<u>Exfoliate your skin gently 2-3 times a week</u>

If your skin tends to get flaky or uneven,

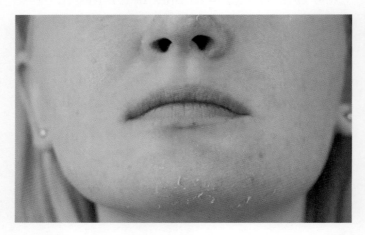

A little gentle exfoliation can help. However, don't do it every day or use harsh scrubs, since this can damage your skin and even lead to breakouts. Apply a gentle exfoliating wash, such as an oatmeal-based exfoliant, and you can well make this yourself. The ingredients for making the oatmeal-based exfoliant are:

1. Oatmeal
2. Coconut oil
3. Baking soda
4. sugar

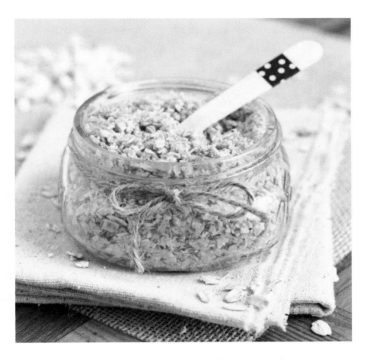

You should apply this with your fingertips, Use small, gentle, circular motions. Rinse the exfoliant away with warm water when you're done.

If you have really sensitive skin, talk to a dermatologist about dermaplaning. This procedure involves gently shaving the skin with a razor to remove fine hairs and dead skin cells; it also helps reduce the appearance of acne scars or other skin imperfections.

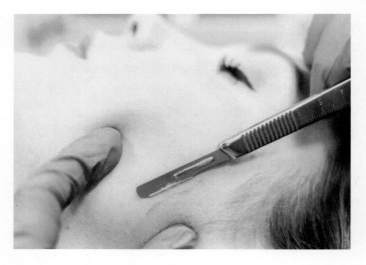

It's gentler than most forms of exfoliation, including scrubs and chemical peels.

Moisturize your skin whenever you shower or wash your face

Bathing, showering, or washing your face can all dry out your skin. To keep your skin happy, soft, and hydrated, put on moisturizer as soon as you're done washing, while your skin is still slightly damp. If you have very dry skin, you may need to moisturize it several times a day. Your hands are especially prone to dryness, since they get a lot of exposure to the elements and must be washed frequently. Try to remember to moisturize your hands any time you wash them.

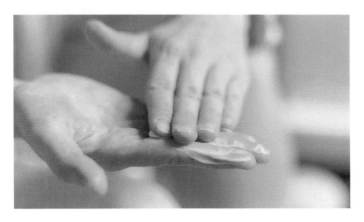

Soothe skin with virgin coconut oil

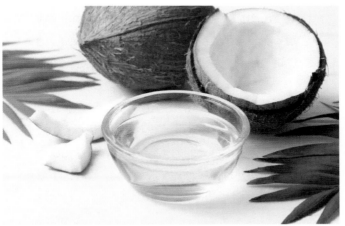

Coconut oil has anti-inflammatory antioxidant, and healing properties. But using coconut oil on your face may not work for every skin type. Do not use if you have allergies to coconut, if you're able to apply it without irritation, it can be used in a number of ways. You can use coconut oil to take off makeup, soothe your skin barrier and promote dewy-looking skin that's healthy below the surface layer. Research Source shows that coconut oil is a good moisturizer. Try massaging a small amount of coconut oil onto your face. Let it soak in for a few minutes before washing off with your normal cleanser.

Use aloe vera to keep skin strong and healthy

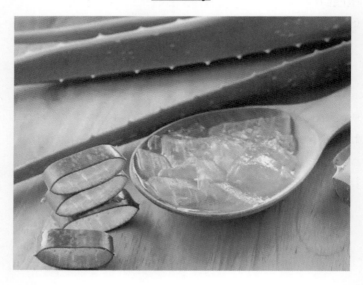

Aloe vera has healing properties and may stimulate new cell growth. It also soothes and moisturizes without clogging pores. Using aloe vera after you've washed your face each day may give your skin that healthy glow.

It's possible to be allergic to aloe vera. Test it first by rubbing a small amount on your forearm and if there's no reaction in 24 hours, it should be safe to use.

Drink more water

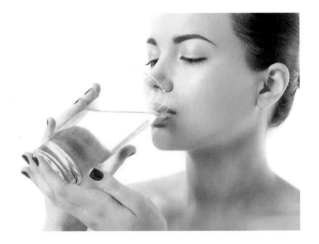

Your skin is made up of cells that need water to function well. The connection to drinking water and having healthy skin is still ongoing, but at least one 2015 study concluded there's a strong link between drinking more water and having healthier skin. Aim for at least eight 8-ounce glasses of water per day.

Find ways to manage stress

When we're stressed or anxious, our bodies release a hormone called cortisol. This hormone activates our flight or fight response (which is a good thing!) but constant stress keeps this response on fatigued overdrive (yep, a bad thing). Specifically to our skin, increased levels of cortisol can cause us to lose our glow by diminishing the skin's ability to retain moisture and encouraging an overproduction of oils.

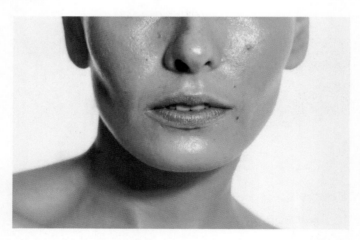

- it causes high levels of cortisol

- puts a damper on your skin's moisture levels, causing dryness and a grey, dull look
- causes a rebound production of oil, which can lead to acne

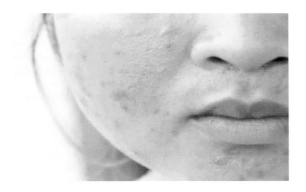

- Premature wrinkle and line development

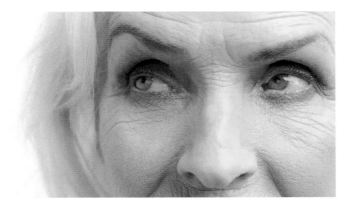

- Redness and inflammation

- inflame and acerbate skin conditions like rosacea, eczema, and psoriasis

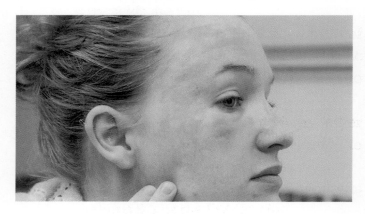

- If that wasn't enough, when you feel anxious or worried, you might notice redness or puffiness in your face. This is a result of increased blood flow, such as dilated blood vessels right underneath the surface of your skin.

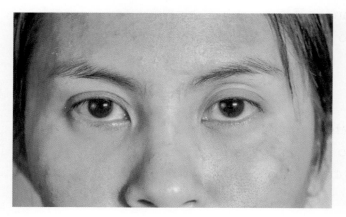

Exercise

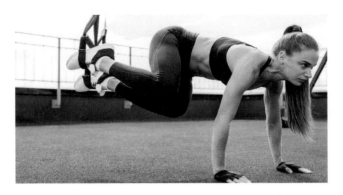

We all know that getting our sweat on is great for our entire body, but it also has some skin benefits as well. When we move, we circulate our blood which carries oxygen and nutrients to all of our cells. Not only does this provide an instant glow, but it also helps our skin to repair itself faster. Another perk to exercise is it helps to reduce stress and, in turn, reduce cortisol levels.

Sleep

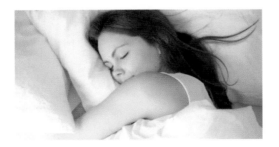

Beauty sleep is the real deal! While we slumber our bodies heal and regenerate cells. Sleep decreases the stress hormone cortisol which is responsible for skin discoloration, thinning skin, and stretch marks.

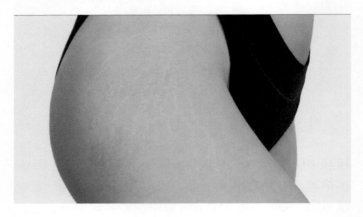

For the good stuff, sleep also increases the sleep hormone melatonin which acts as an antioxidantto fights fine lines, wrinkles, and skin cancer. While snoozing we also produce new collagen which helps keep our face looking plump and wrinkle-free. Last but not least, we produce a large amount of human growth hormone while we sleep which helps to repair the damage we encounter on a daily basis.

CHAPTER TWO

Organic Facial Treatment

Facials are basically any kind of skin care treatment specifically meant for the face; it involves massage, exfoliation, creams, extractions and facial masks and is common in salons and spas.

There are many health and beauty companies that focus on processing essential natural ingredients used for facial treatments, and these ingredients provide facial improvement and enhance the smoothness of the face.

However, there are natural ways by which the hidden toxins, harmful ingredients and chemical effects on the outermost parts of the body specifically the face can be treated.

Just the same way salons do facial treatment with commercially obtained products; you can as well apply the natural ingredients following the procedures below to bring out the real beauty in you.

Listed are some of the natural ingredients that can be used for facial treatments;

1. Apple Cider Vinegar

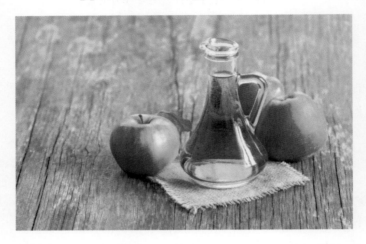

2. Coconut Oil

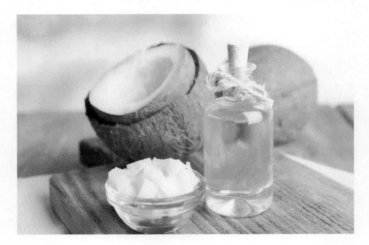

3. Avocado

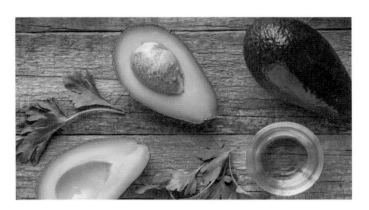

4. Aloe Vera

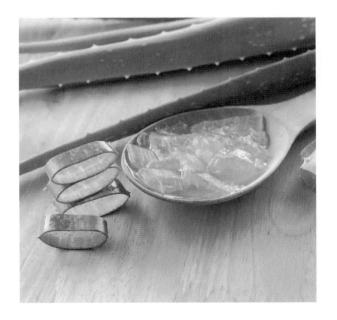

5. Argan Oil

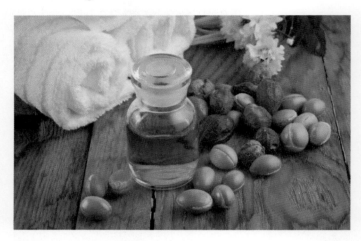

6. Sea Salt

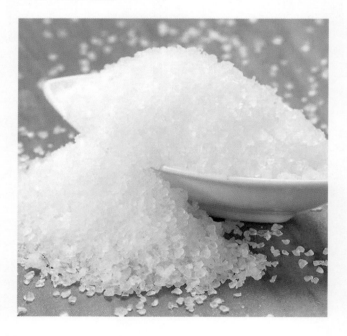

7. Tea Tree Oil

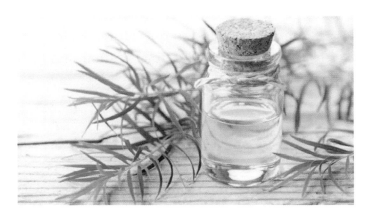

8. Lemon Essential Oil

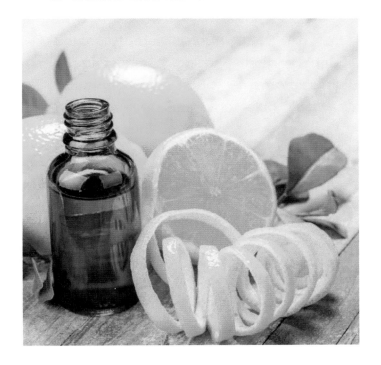

9. Castor Oil

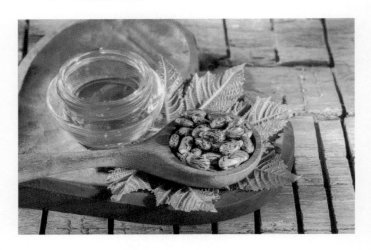

10. Shea Butter

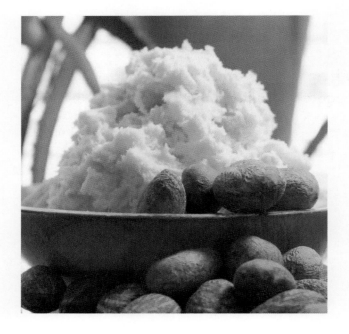

11. Almond Oil

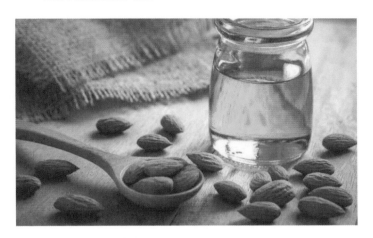

12. Jojoba

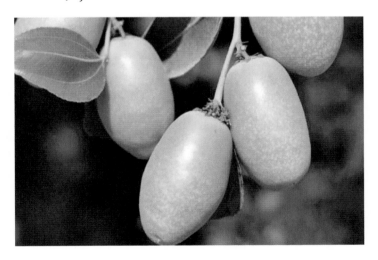

13. Raw Honey

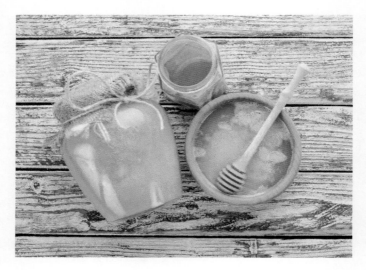

Facial Cleansing

Before you do your facial cleansing, you have to wash your face in order to remove your makeup completely. Some makeup such as mascara, concealer and foundation can be washed off totally by dissolving with an oil-based cream and washing off with lukewarm water.

Once you are done with washing off the makeup, follow the steps provided below to cleanse the face.

1. Get a teaspoon full of castor oil

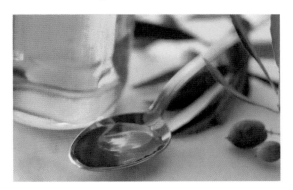

2. Mixed into one-quarter of almond or coconut oil
3. Rub it thoroughly on the face and after some seconds wash it out with lukewarm water to clean out impurities on the face.

Facial Scrubbing/Exfoliating

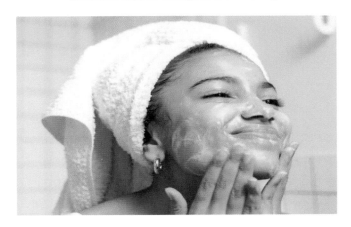

This involves the stage of removing the dead cells on the skin which also includes the remaining dirt that was not removed during the cleansing process and is advised to do this at least once a week.

One good thing about this natural facial exfoliating is that the ingredients are obtainable everywhere and they are quite inexpensive and works even better

There are several methods for exfoliating which includes but is not limited to the options below;

A. 1 tablespoon of organic sugar cane or granulated sugar

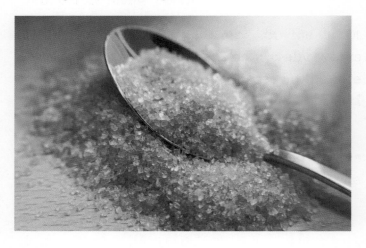

B. 1 to 2 drops of lemon orange or lavender oil

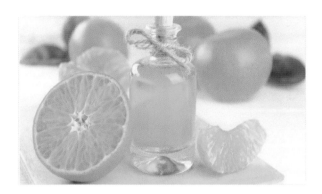

C. And a little water to make the mixture a bit thick.

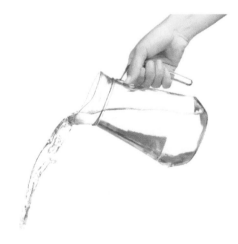

- Mix them together in a neat container using the tip of your finger.

- Rub nicely on the face and be careful in order not to penetrate into the eyes.
- Then rinse with cold water and dry with a towel after 20 minutes.

Alternative natural ingredients for scrubbing are

A. 1 tablespoon of olive oil

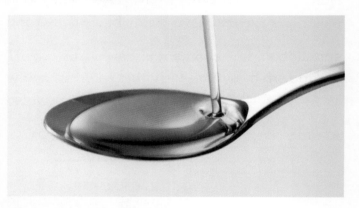

B. 1 tablespoon of raw/local honey

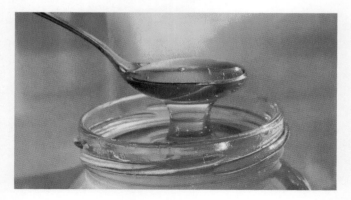

C. Half fresh lemon

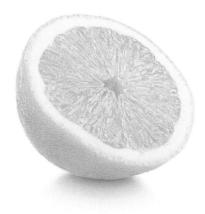

D. Half granulated sugar

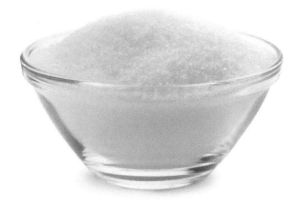

Then mix

- Apply and clean or get 2 tablespoons of sugar and 1 tablespoon of coconut oil mix together.
- Clean the face very well then apply it on the face and neck area smoothly.
- After I minute, rinse with warm water and dry it off

Facial Massage

Method One

This method is also another natural treatment that can be applied on the face to make to look more beautiful and captivating. There are several ingredients and their different method of blending for facial massage.

A. Get one teaspoon full of aloe vera gel freshly extracted from the leaves.

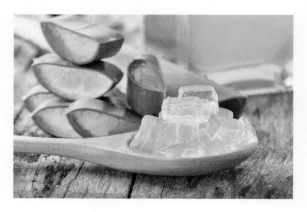

B. A small piece of ripe paw-paw

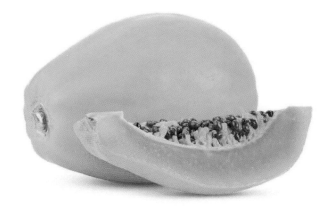

C. One slice of seedless orange

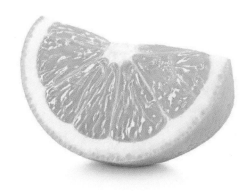

D. And one piece of strawberry or its alternative (3-4 grapes)

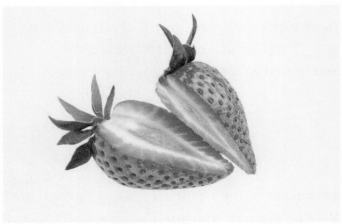

Blending: Use a blender to mix up the ingredients to obtain fine pulpy cream for your daily facial massage.

Method Two

Facial massage can as well be done using

A. lemon juice

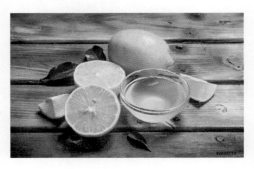

B. Tomato juice

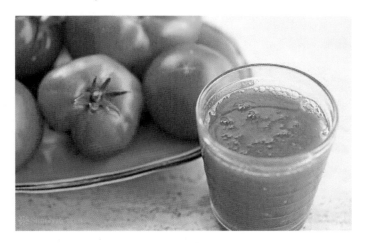

C. Glycerin

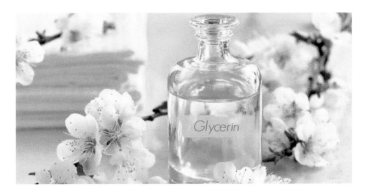

Mix the same quantity of the three ingredients together and apply gently on the face for massage to remove dirt.

Method Three

Another is orange facial massage which is done by boiling peeled orange slices in little quantity of water for up to 10 minutes.

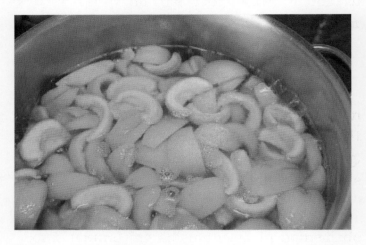

Allow it to cool then sieve it gently and use for facial massage.

Method Four

Steaming

Steaming is another method of facial treatment with natural ingredients. It helps to relax the facial skin and give it a beautiful styling look. Additionally, it allows the skin to release a wide variety of toxins and carcinogens.

This can simply be done using this method:

A. Boil a clean water

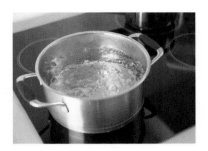

B. Then place a towel over your head to close to the pot of hot water so that the steam reaches the face quickly. Do not put your face very close to the hot water.

C. Then lean over the pot or bowl for 5 to 10 minutes to steam your face. Blow into the pot from time to time to let out more vapour as the steam gets cold.

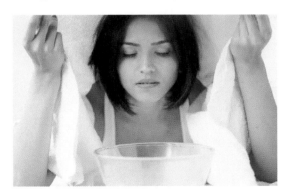

Face Mask

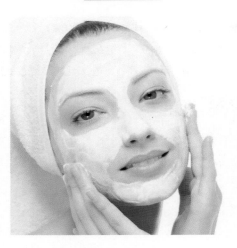

Face masking is a very important treatment that helps to tighten pores on the face, hydrate the skin of the face, remove impurities, tone the skin, nourish, refresh and then keep skin pores neat so as to allow penetration of moisturizing ingredients to penetrate well into the skin and should be done on weekly basis (twice as the case may be).

Before doing this, make sure that you have steamed your face so that it can absorb some nutrition involved in face masking. There are several natural methods but you can choose one depending on what you want and your skin type;

Method One

Application of egg white is the simplest

A. Break an egg, extract the egg white, whisk with a fork until it foams very well

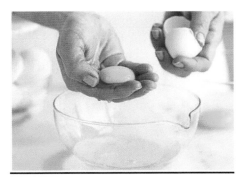

B. With the use of your fingers apply the egg white on the face.
C. Immediately after the application, place tissue paper on the face to make a mask then leave it for an hour.

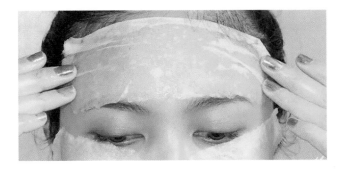

Then peel the mask and wash your face with cold water.

Other natural ingredients and their methods of application for face mask are

Method Two

Cinnamon and honey:

A. Get 1 teaspoon full of honey

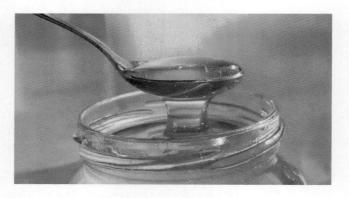

B. And 2 teaspoons of cinnamon

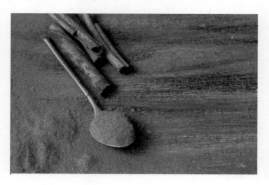

- Mix until it foams then apply on the face and leave it overnight
- Wash the next morning with warm water

Method Three

Banana, lemon, and honey

A. Get 1 teaspoon of honey

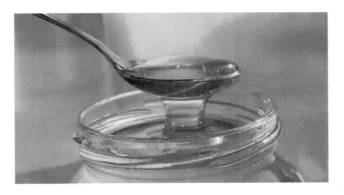

B. Up to 10 drops of lemon juice

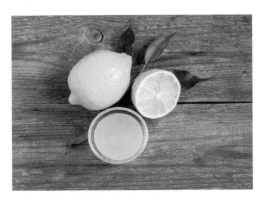

C. A banana

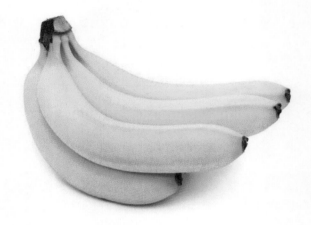

D. And a tissue

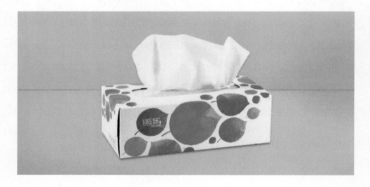

- Peel the banana and mash very well in a clean bowl.
- Add exactly 10 drops of lemon and one spoon of honey.

- Stir very well until it becomes very silky then rub on the face and allow it for just 20 minutes.
- Wash with cold water and dry with your tissue.

Method Four

Egg white, avocados, and lemon juice

A. Egg White

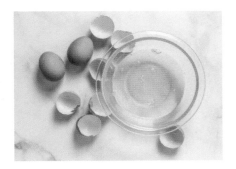

B. Avocado

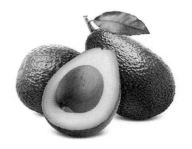

- Mash half quantity of avocado pulp in a neat small basin.
- Add lemon juice and egg white and blend very well until it becomes smooth.
- Apply on the face, leave it for 20 minutes then wash with warm water and dry your face.

<u>Whitening Facial at Home:</u>

Whitening facial is one of the methods that can be used to tone and brighten the complexion. It helps to remove dead cells, skin darkening, acne, premature ageing and dullness on the face.

Some natural ingredients used in homemade products for skin whitening are

A. Milk

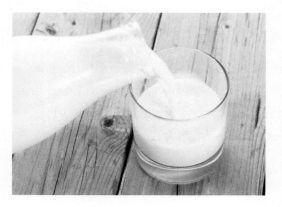

B. Honey

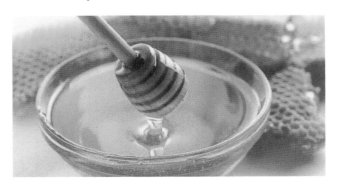

C. Papaya

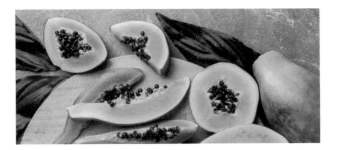

D. sandalwood powder

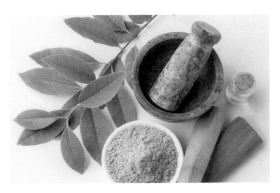

E. And rose Water

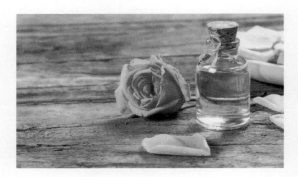

Do not forget that before applying a facial treatment that the face has to be washed as we explained earlier. In fact, before you apply whitening facial ensure that your face has undergone any of the tips listed above.

At this juncture, you can prepare your natural whitening facial pack which takes a few steps and ingredients such as sandalwood powder, rose water or milk.

For Dry Skin

- Get a mixture of 2 teaspoonfuls of milk and sandalwood powder.
- Apply it on the thick layer of the face.
- Allow mixture to dry on the face before washing it out.

- Then apply some toning cream on the face after you must have washed the whitening pack.

For Oily Skin:

- Mix 2 teaspoonful of sandalwood powder with rose water very well in a clean bowl then follow the same steps used for dry skin.

Homemade Chemical Peel Recipe

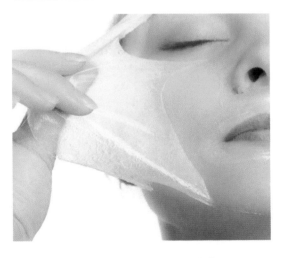

Peels is another kind of natural face treatment that helps to improve and smoothen the texture of the skin.

Facial peeling removes the outermost layers of the skin and the results which occur as wound healing is what regenerates new tissues and eventually peels off the dead skin.

When naturally made chemical peels are used, the regenerated skin is usually smoother and less wrinkled compared to the old skin.

The ingredients needed to make this natural chemical are:

1. One small seeded cucumber

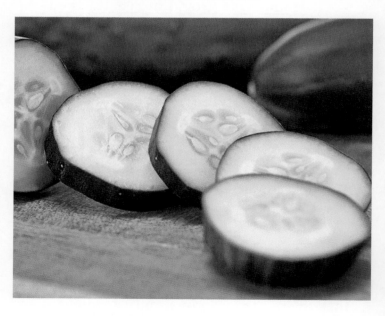

2. One package or tablespoon of unflavored gelatin,

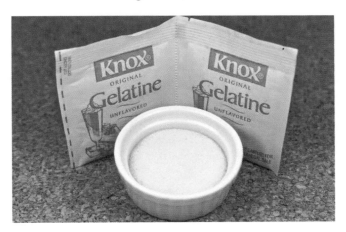

3. Few drops of a natural meat tenderizer or half teaspoon of powdered meat tenderizer,

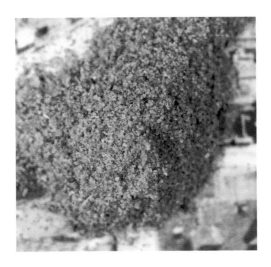

4. one dash ground of cinnamon

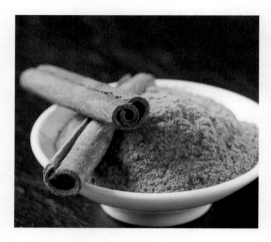

5. And water

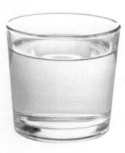

- Put the cucumber inside a neat container

- And sprinkle with the gelatin. If it fails to dissolve, add water in it.
- Inside the mixture prepared in step I above, sprinkle meat tenderizer and cinnamon, then stir up the mixture combine very well while the gelatin dissolves and become pasty.
- Spread the mixture on the face and allow for 15 to 20 minutes to dry very well.
- When it must have dried well on the face, start from the jaw to peel slowly from the face.

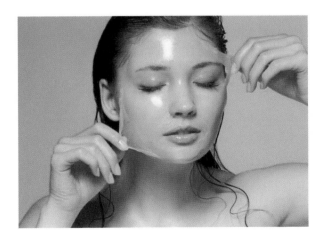

- Rinse off and apply moisturizer.

The face is a sensitive part of the body and is always exposed to sunlight and unfriendly atmosphere, so it is important to apply natural ingredients for the facial treatment at least once in a week in order to maintain a smooth and moisturized face

And these natural ingredients will save you unnecessary expenses of buying packaged chemicals from the market which may react to your skin and damage the face.

Any natural ingredient you mix for the face must be used on the back of your hand or any other part of the body and be left there for few seconds to ensure that it doesn't react to your skin before using it on the face.

Conclusively, facials are one of the most essential skin care regimens as it really works down deep to reach into the pores on the face to open them up, make the face smoother and prettier.

But one has to be mindful of the kind of face wipes or substances used in cleaning up the face before applying the natural ingredients.

Note that most wipes we use are packed with loads of chemicals which might even counter our beauty treatment.

CHAPTER THREE

Facial Extraction

This involves the act of squeezing a giant spot or pimples on the face.

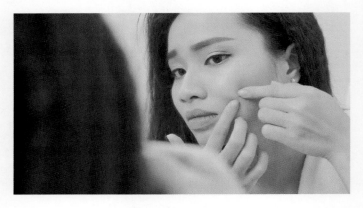

It's another facial treatment which most of us do but we actually do this in a very wrong way.

People suffer from chronic acne which must have caused inflammation on the face as a result of popping the pimples in a wrong way. Provided below are some important measures of doing this.

A. Steam the skin to get softened and clear out some bacteria or toxins on the skin.

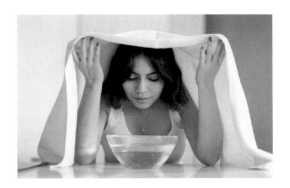

B. Apply a bioactive purifying face mask on the areas where the face has been affected with acne, rinse off with warm water after the mask must have dried up on the face area.

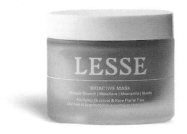

C. Use medical gloves or round tissue paper round the index finger before popping pimples on the face as bare fingers add the different strain of bacteria to the blemishes on the face.

D. Place the tip of the finger in a c-shaped form into the tissue and break the pimples.

E. Clean with little hydrogen peroxide

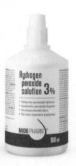

F. And apply acne treatment cream on the surface area when it must have stopped oozing out fluid or blood.

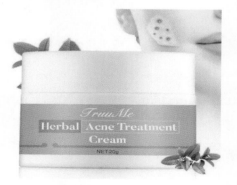

CHAPTER FOUR

Food\Fruit That Nourishes The Skin

Nutrition is important for health. An unhealthy diet can damage your metabolism, cause weight gain, and even damage organs, such as your heart and liver. But what you eat also affects another organ, your skin.

As scientists learn more about diet and the body, it's increasingly clear that what you eat can significantly affect the health and aging of your skin.

Take a look at 12 of the best foods for keeping your skin healthy.

1. Fatty fish

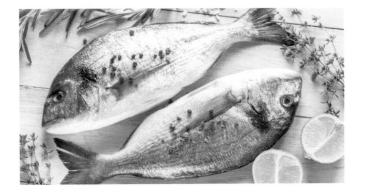

Fatty fish such as

Salmon

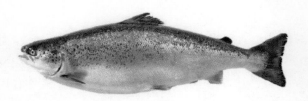

Mackerel

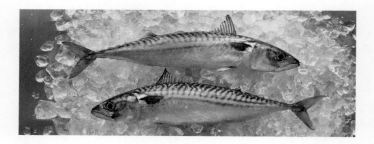

And herring

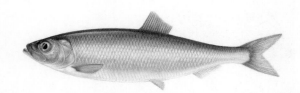

A. Fatty fish are excellent foods for healthy skin. They're rich sources of omega-3 fatty acids, which are important for maintaining skin health.

B. Omega 3 fatty acids are necessary to help keep skin thick, supple, and moisturized. In fact, an omega 3 fatty acid deficiency can cause dry skin.

C. The omega 3 fats in fish reduce inflammation, which can cause redness and acne. They can even make your skin less sensitive to the sun's harmful UV rays.

D. Some studies show that fish oil supplements may help fight inflammatory and autoimmune conditions affecting your skin, such as psoriasis and lupus.

E. Fatty fish is also a source of vitamin E, one of the most important antioxidants for your skin.

F. Getting enough vitamin E is essential for helping protect your skin against damage from free radicals and inflammation.

G. This type of seafood is also a source of high quality protein, which is needed for maintaining the strength and integrity of your skin.

H. Lastly, fish provides zinc a mineral vital for regulating the following:

- Inflammation
- Overall skin health
- The production of new skin cells
- Zinc deficiency can lead to skin inflammation, lesions, and delayed wound healing.

Summary

Fatty types of fish like salmon contain omega-3 fatty acids that can reduce inflammation and keep your skin moisturized. They're also a good source of high quality protein, vitamin E, and zinc.

2. **Avocados**

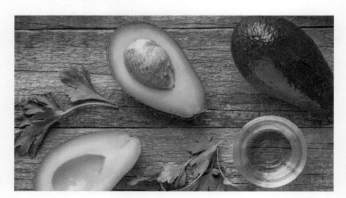

Avocados are high in healthy fats. These fats benefit many functions in your body, including the health of your skin

A. Getting enough of these fats is essential to help keep skin flexible and moisturized.

B. One study involving over 700 women found that a high intake of total fat specifically the types of healthy fats found in avocados was associated with more supple, springy skin.

C. Preliminary evidence also shows that avocados contain compounds that may help protect your skin from sun damage. UV damage to your skin can cause wrinkles and other signs of aging.

D. Avocados are also a good source of vitamin E, which is an important antioxidant that helps protect your skin from oxidative damage. Most Americans don't get enough vitamin E through their diet.

E. Interestingly, vitamin E seems to be more effective when combined with vitamin C.

F. Vitamin C is also essential for healthy skin. Your skin needs it to create collagen, which is the main structural protein that keeps your skin strong and healthy.

G. Vitamin C deficiency is rare these days, but common symptoms include dry, rough, and scaly skin that tends to bruise easily.

H. Vitamin C is also an antioxidant that helps protect your skin from oxidative damage caused by the sun and the environment, which can lead to signs of aging.

I. A 100-gram serving, or about 1/2 an avocado, provides 14% of the Daily Value (DV) for vitamin E and 11% of the DV for vitamin C.

Summary

Avocados are high in beneficial fats and contain vitamins E and C, which are important for healthy skin. They also pack compounds that may protect your skin from sun damage.

3. <u>Walnuts</u>

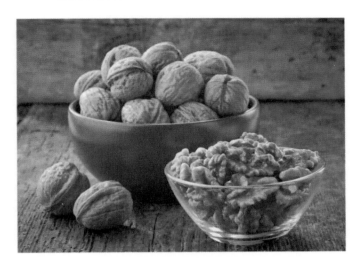

Walnuts have many characteristics that make them an excellent food for healthy skin.

A. They're a good source of essential fatty acids, which are fats that your body cannot make itself. In fact, they're richer than most other nuts in both omega-3 and omega-6 fatty acids.

B. A diet too high in omega-6 fats may promote inflammation, including inflammatory conditions of your skin like psoriasis. On the other hand, omega 3 fats reduce inflammation in your body including in your skin.

C. While omega 6 fatty acids are plentiful in the Western diet, sources of omega 3 fatty acids are rare.

D. Because walnuts contain a good ratio of these fatty acids, they may help fight the potential inflammatory response to excessive omega 6.

E. What's more, walnuts contain other nutrients that your skin needs to function properly and stay healthy.

F. One ounce (28 grams) of walnuts contains 8% of the DV for zinc.

G. Zinc is essential for your skin to function properly as a barrier. It's also necessary for wound healing and combating both bacteria and inflammation.

H. Walnuts also provide small amounts of the antioxidants vitamin E and selenium, in addition to 4–5 grams of protein per ounce (28 grams).

Summary

Walnuts are a good source of essential fats, zinc, vitamin E, selenium and protein all of which are nutrients your skin needs to stay healthy.

4. Sunflower seeds

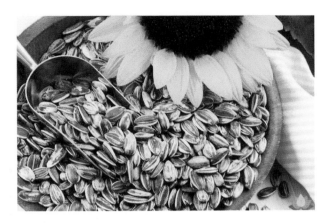

In general, nuts and seeds are good sources of skin boosting nutrients.

Sunflower seeds are an excellent example.

A. One ounce (28 grams) of sunflower seeds packs 49% of the DV for vitamin E, 41% of the DV for selenium, 14% of the DV for zinc, and 5.5 grams of protein.

Summary

Sunflower seeds are an excellent source of nutrients, including vitamin E, which is an important antioxidant for the skin.

5. <u>Sweet potatoes</u>

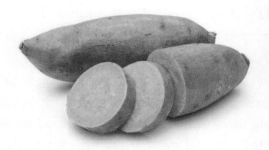

Beta carotene is a nutrient found in plants. It functions as provitamin A, which means it can be converted into vitamin A in your body. Beta carotene is found in oranges and vegetables such as carrots, spinach, and sweet potatoes.

Sweet potatoes are an excellent source one 1/2-cup (100-gram) serving of baked sweet potato contains enough beta carotene to provide more than six times the DV of vitamin A.

A. Carotenoids like beta carotene help keep your skin healthy by acting as a natural sunblock.

B. When consumed, this antioxidant is incorporated into your skin and helps protect your skin cells from sun exposure. This may help prevent sunburn, cell death, and dry, wrinkled skin.
C. Interestingly, high amounts of beta carotene may also add a warm, orange color to your skin, contributing to an overall healthier appearance.

Summary

Sweet potatoes are an excellent source of beta carotene, which acts as a natural sunblock and may protect your skin from sun damage.

6. **Red or yellow bell peppers**

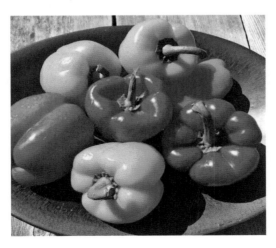

Like sweet potatoes, bell peppers are an excellent source of beta carotene, which your body converts into vitamin A.

    A. One cup (149 grams) of chopped red bell pepper contains the equivalent of 156% of the DV for vitamin A.

    B. They're also one of the best sources of vitamin C. This vitamin is necessary for creating the protein collagen, which keeps skin firm and strong.

    C. A single cup (149 grams) of bell pepper provides an impressive 211% of the DV for vitamin C.

    D. A large observational study involving women linked eating plenty of vitamin C to a reduced risk of wrinkled and dry skin with age.

Summary

Bell peppers contain plenty of beta carotene and vitamin C — both of which are important antioxidants for your skin. Vitamin C is also necessary to create collagen, the structural protein that keeps your skin strong.

7. <u>Broccoli</u>

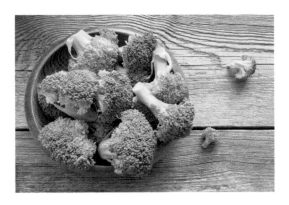

A. Broccoli is full of many vitamins and minerals important for skin health, including zinc, vitamin A, and vitamin C.

B. It also contains lutein, a carotenoid that works like beta carotene. Lutein helps protect your skin from oxidative damage, which can cause your skin to become dry and wrinkled.

C. But broccoli florets also pack a special compound called sulforaphane, which boasts some impressive potential benefits. It may even have anti-cancer effects, including on some types of skin cancer.

D. Sulforaphane is likewise a powerful protective agent against sun damage. It works in two ways: neutralizing harmful free radicals and switching on other protective systems in your body.

E. In laboratory tests, sulforaphane reduced the number of skin cells UV light killed by as much as 29%, with protection lasting up to 48 hours.

F. Evidence suggests sulforaphane may also help maintain collagen levels in your skin.

Summary

Broccoli is a good source of vitamins, minerals, and carotenoids that are important for skin health. It also contains sulforaphane, which may help prevent skin cancer and protect your skin from sunburn.

8. Tomatoes

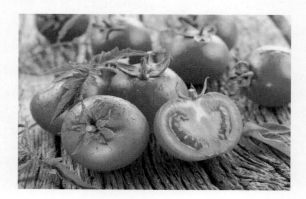

Tomatoes are a great source of vitamin C and contain all of the major carotenoids, including lycopene.

A. Beta carotene, lutein, and lycopene have been shown to protect your skin against damage from the sun. They may also help prevent wrinkling.
B. Because tomatoes are rich in carotenoids, they're an excellent food for maintaining healthy skin.
C. Consider pairing carotenoid-rich foods like tomatoes with a source of fat, such as cheese or olive oil. Fat increases your absorption of carotenoids.

Summary

Tomatoes are a good source of vitamin C and all of the major carotenoids, especially lycopene. These carotenoids protect your skin from sun damage and may help prevent wrinkling.

9. <u>Soy</u>

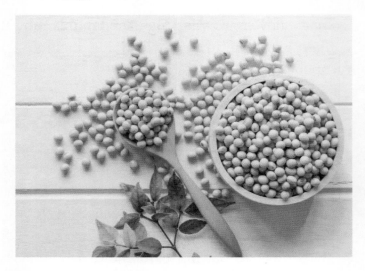

Soy contains isoflavones, a category of plant compounds that can either mimic or block estrogen in your body.

A. Isoflavones may benefit several parts of your body, including your skin.
B. One small study involving middle-aged women found that eating soy isoflavones every day for 8–12 weeks reduced fine wrinkles and improved skin elasticity.
C. In postmenopausal women, soy may also improve skin dryness and increase

collagen, which helps keep your skin smooth and strong.

D. These isoflavones not only help to protect the cells inside your body from damage but also your skin from UV radiation — which may reduce the risk of some skin cancers.

<u>Summa</u>

Soy contains isoflavones, which have been shown to improve wrinkles, collagen, and skin elasticity and skin dryness, as well as protect your skin from UV damage.

10. <u>Dark chocolate</u>

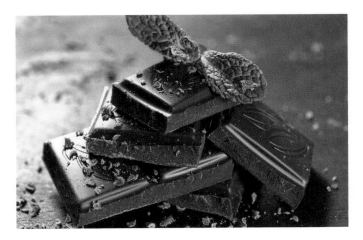

If you need one more reason to eat chocolate, here it is: The effects of cocoa on your skin are pretty phenomenal.

A. After 6–12 weeks of consuming a cocoa powder high in antioxidants each day, participants in one study experienced thicker, more hydrated skin.

B. Their skin was also less rough and scaly, less sensitive to sunburn, and had better blood flow which brings more nutrients to your skin.

C. Another study found that eating 20 grams of high-antioxidant dark chocolate per day could allow your skin to withstand over twice as much UV radiation before burning, compared with eating low-antioxidant chocolate.

D. Several other studies have observed similar results, including improvements in the appearance of wrinkles. However, keep in mind that at least one study didn't find significant effects.

E. Make sure to choose dark chocolate with at least 70% cocoa to maximize the benefits and keep added sugar to a minimum.

Summary

Cocoa contains antioxidants that may protect your skin against sunburn. These antioxidants may also improve wrinkles, skin thickness, hydration, blood flow, and skin texture.

11. Green tea

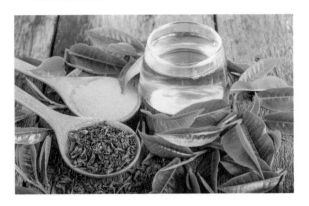

Green tea may help protect your skin from damage and aging.

A. The powerful compounds found in green tea are called catechins and work to improve the health of your skin in several ways.
B. Like several other antioxidant-containing foods, green tea can help protect your skin against sun damage.

C. One 12-week study involving 60 women found that drinking green tea daily could reduce redness from sun exposure by up to 25%.
D. Green tea also improved the moisture, roughness, thickness, and elasticity of their skin.
E. While green tea is a great choice for healthy skin, you may want to avoid drinking your tea with milk, as there's evidence that milk could reduce the effect of green tea's antioxidants.

Summary

The catechins found in green tea are powerful antioxidants that can protect your skin against sun damage and reduce redness, as well as improve its hydration, thickness and elasticity.

12. Red grapes

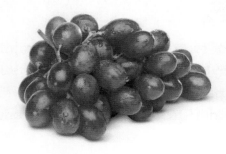

Red grapes are famous for containing resveratrol, a compound that comes from the skin of red grapes.

A. Resveratrol is credited with a wide range of health benefits, among them is reducing the effects of aging.

B. Test-tube studies suggest it may also help slow the production of harmful free radicals, which damage skin cells and cause signs of aging.

C. This beneficial compound is also found in red wine. Unfortunately, there's not much evidence that the amount of resveratrolyou get from a glass of red wine is enough to affect your skin.

D. And since red wine is an alcoholic beverage, there are negative effects to drinking it in excess. It's not recommended to start drinking red wine just because of its potential health benefits. Instead, you should increase your intake of red grapes and berries.

Summary

Resveratrol, the famous antioxidant found in red grapes, may slow your skin's aging process by impairing harmful free radicals that damage your skin.

CHAPTER FIVE

Why And How You Should Protect Your Skin

1. Limit your time in the sun

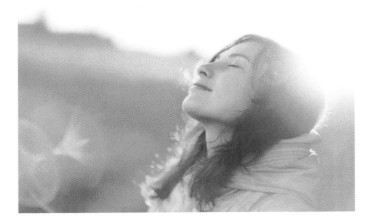

Yes, use sunscreen but for the non product part of it: it's time to play hide and seek, An estimated 90 percent of skin aging is caused by the sun, specifically for folks with lighter skin and not to mention the even scarier risk of skin cancer. Considering that's a pretty huge number, it's best to limit your sun exposure or seek shade when hanging out.

Don't forget to protect your eyes where you can't apply sunscreen too! Squinting doesn't exactly protect your eyes and if you insist on doing the peering exercise, you may end up developing more lines and wrinkles around your eye and forehead area

2. **<u>Opting out of sugar</u>**

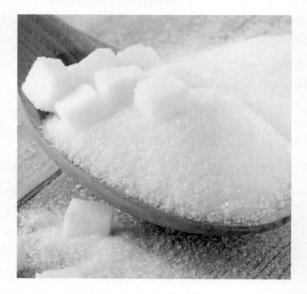

Sometimes the skin takes a while to catch up to how we felt or what we ate last week. If your energy source is primarily added sugar and refined carbohydrates, you might start seeing the effects of that on your skin.

After all, too much of one thing strains the body and skin. Too much exfoliating acids may strip your skin's protective barrier, just like too much sugar may cause a surge in insulin (the hormone produced by the pancreas that regulates the amount of sugar in the blood), and inflammation. This process produces an enzyme that attaches to collagen fibers breaking them down and causing them to lose strength and flexibility.

If you're noticing your skin becoming more vulnerable to sun damage, a loss of elasticity, acne production, and more arrivals the wrinkles and lines department, check in with yourself: what's driving your diet and can you take back control?

Addressing stress, for example, may help revive the brain energy you need for creating home cooked meals. Studies show that your acne and/or rosacea gets better or worse based on what you eat, so it might be diet related as well.

Insulin surges may put your oil glands in overdrive, creating a breeding ground for acne to form. Fortunately, there are products to counteract that so if sugar and refined carbs are staples to your diet, eat away, and rely on products instead!

3. <u>Avoid being around cigarette smoke</u>

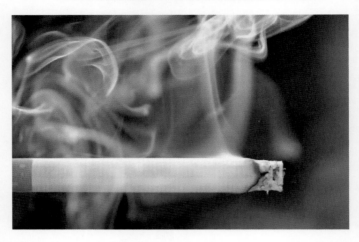

When tobacco is heated via cigarettes or even, yes, vaping it releases free radicals that damage the DNA of skin cells. This results in the breakdown of collagen and elastin.

It also constricts blood vessels which deplete the skin of much needed oxygen, vitamins, and nutrients. When that puff of toxic smoke is exhaled it hits the skin on the face and can cause blackheads, particularly around the mouth and cheek areas.

Over time this leads to accelerated aging, dehydration, dark circles, broken blood vessels, and an overall dull looking complexion. Studies also indicate that smokers heal slower than non smokers. That means when you do get a pimple it can take longer to heal which can lead to post inflammatory hyper pigmentation.

Printed in Great Britain
by Amazon

40190847R00050